Get Healthy:
The Middle-Aged
Man's Survival Guide

Simple step by step methods to regain your good health

ZACKARY RICHARDS

Ari Publishing

Get Healthy-The Middle-Aged Man's Survival Guide was written by Zackary Richards

Disclaimer

Any person embarking on a new diet or health regimen should always consult their physician first. The author is NOT A Licensed Medical Professional and although the health plan outlined in this book greatly improved his health through changes in diet and exercise, you however, may have other health issues that require the supervision of a licensed professional, especially if you have food allergies, physical disabilities or on multiple medications. Never stop taking prescribed medications without consulting your doctor.

Hello and Welcome

If you're reading this you likely want to get your health back, lose those extra pounds, add a little muscle and not run out of breath every time you climb the stairs.

If so, I'm your guy.

But first let me point out that <u>I AM NOT A DOCTOR,</u> nor am I a nutritionist or dietician. Common sense dictates that before beginning any diet regimen or exercise program you discuss it with your physician. I am merely a writer who found himself in an overweight, deteriorating physical condition who decided to find the most effective methods of getting my health back.

I knew that if I didn't take action I'd either wind up in an early grave or become one of these morbidly obese people you seen riding around big box stores in those motorized carts with a tank of oxygen on their lap.

So I tried all the latest diets and weight loss programs and the horrific exercise regimens that came with some hulking imbecile standing over me shouting, "Give me TEN MORE!"

Most of the time none of that stuff worked, and when it did, I gained the weight back in a few months.

Sound familiar?

What I'm going to show you won't involve any misery, starvation or exhaustion.

I'll simply show you what to eat and what to do physically to regain your health and start feeling good again.

And I'll show you how to do it in ways that you can easily incorporate into your daily life.

This is no Fitnessinsane.com. Frankly, I get exhausted just watching those people.

So let's look at the other side of the spectrum.

Planet Fitness is a place where you go to exercise. They don't like being called a gym because that word intimidates people. Reminds them of over-muscled lunk heads showing off and making everyone else feel uncomfortable and inferior.

Their clever marketing campaign established them as the place where regular people can get back into shape. No lunks, no body-builders. Simple, easy, not intimidating. It became very successful.

It was a great idea and I decided to emulate it regarding diet and health.

The problem with most of today's diets is that they are put together by super-healthy fanatics whose passion is fitness. Like the intimidating body builders, they go too far. They push the idea that any food that isn't overloaded with vitamins and nutrients, and doesn't smell and taste like swamp grass is SLOWLY KILLING YOU!

No it isn't.

These people have no idea what it's like to be middle-aged and so they create diets that make demands best suited for a guy in his twenties, not his fifties. Plus these diets require too much time and effort. My passion is not fitness. I'm not looking to run a marathon. Or win a weight lifting contest. I don't need rock-hard abs. I don't need a body mass indicator of under 10%.

Besides if you're lugging around 30-60 or more extra pounds, you're not going to participate in a fitness program whose first step is to do 25 squat-thrusts.

All I want is for my internal machinery to run properly. I want clean filters, unclogged pipes, strong superstructure, fresh fluids, proper ventilation, pressure and temperature.

Following my twice a year physical, I want my doctor to say, "You're fine, everything is working properly, I'll see you in six months.

Another reason most diets fail is the psychology behind it. Nobody wants to go on a diet and, because I am asking you to do something for me, (follow my diet and exercise plan) you inherently feel as if you're doing me a favor. It's human nature. So if the diet plan is too restrictive or demanding, you eventually say to yourself, *Screw this guy, I'm going to eat whatever I want!* Ergo, you have taught me a lesson and your righteous indignation has been satisfied.

And unfortunately you fall back into unhealthy eating habits.

Since this is often the case, I've had to find a way around that. I have to convince you that by eating certain foods and snacks that actually taste good AND are good for you, you won't rebel against the diet and stick with it.

That's it! That's all I need you to do. Just follow it and you will begin to feel better, sleep better and have more energy AND very likely lose weight in the process.

Once you have your health back THEN, you can decide how much more weight you want to lose and how much more exercise you want to do.

Here's another way to look at these harsh restrictive diets.

Imagine you're cruising along in the fast lane, which we will rename the fast FOOD lane. You're eating whatever tastes good and using TUMS or Rolaids to fight off the acid reflux. Life is good.

Then suddenly one of your dashboard warning lights come on. Buzzers sound and alerts flash. In panic you swerve into the middle and then slow lanes causing all kinds of trouble.

Once there, you decrease your speed, drive cautiously and carefully monitor your dashboard for any further signs of trouble.

After a while the warning lights go out and the alerts go quiet. So you tell yourself it was just a one-time glitch and start heading back into the fast FOOD lane again.

Everything is fine for a while then BOOM, the lights come on again and the buzzers sound. You immediately swerve toward the slow lane only this time you cut off a tractor-trailer.

And yes, this is going to hurt.

In simple terms these yo-yo diets damage your body. When you rapidly lose weight then gain it back again your body creates visceral fat. Which is fat stored, not on the waistline, but in between your organs which can affect their efficiency.

However, making realistic moderate changes to your diet over a period of time will strengthen your body internally and boost your immune system, and that is far more important for a middle-aged man than being able to do drop 50 pounds in 6 weeks and do 50 pull ups.

Make sense? If so let me tell you my story so you can decide if I'm a person you want to work with.

Jerry Garcia once said, "When life looks like easy street, there's danger at your door." Which means if you are at a point in your life when everything is going right and everything is working to your advantage, it's a warning that your life is going to go very bad, very soon."

I discovered just how true that saying was on my 45th birthday.

Things *were* good. I had a book publishing contract, a good paying job, an affordable mortgage and a great wife and kids. And on that birthday I was with friends and family. We saw a show, went for a boat ride, ate at a top of the line restaurant, then partied into the wee hours.

I FINALLY had the life I had always wanted!

In the months and years that followed however, it all fell apart at a dizzying rate. The kids went off to college and my wife learned she was going deaf, and, in addition, her particular form of hearing loss could not be helped with hearing aids. As her condition progressed she came to hate her job because she couldn't hear people walking up behind her, nor hear them call her name and she was startled every time someone tapped her on the shoulder. So her co-workers ostracized and avoided her.

And over time she had come to resent me because I, admittedly, was trying to avoid talking to her as well, because when we did talk, I had to repeat what I said over and over and too often, she still misheard or misunderstood.

Yes, deafness is a terrible condition.

My wife and I could no longer go to the movies because she couldn't hear the dialogue. When we'd watch TV, we had to keep the closed captioning on, and when she couldn't read it fast enough, she's ask me what they said and I'd miss the next few minutes of the show while explaining it to her.

As her hearing loss progressed, she'd claim I was intentionally mumbling, or that I was shouting. Or quote me as saying things I had never said, but she believed she heard.

It's often said that the key to a successful marriage is communication. That's true. A great marriage that had lasted over two decades was in serious trouble.

And to top it off, during that time I had a series of health problems of my own including a cancer scare. The Great Recession was gearing up and my fellow employees were being let go at a furious rate. I mistakenly thought I was safe because my department was still profitable.

I lasted longer than most but come early 2011 I was out of a job. Fortunately I had a publishing deal and the royalties from my first book were pretty good. My second had been put on the fast track so I figured the combined royalties would solve any money issues.

But then my second book was delayed, then delayed again. Then I learned my publisher was in financial trouble.

A week later they closed down.

It was during this time when my wife filed for divorce and a lengthy legal battle ensued. And it was during that time that I went into a serious depression. I didn't want to come home so I stuffed my face at fast food joints. And when I was home, I'd lock myself in my office with a pack of cigarettes, coffee and a small fridge filled with microwavable TV dinners and other very unhealthy crap.

Over a period of 18 months I had ballooned to nearly 300 pounds. I had chronic acid reflux, afib, swollen ankles and fingers, chronic hypertension, shortness of breath, insomnia and anxiety attacks.

When I finally decided to rejoin the land of the living, I saw that the enormousness of the task of getting back into shape. I wasn't sure I could do it.

But I did try.

It just didn't work. And it didn't work because I had become a rage monster and bristled when some trainer started in with that drill sergeant bullshit. And being hungry all the time only made things worse.

Then one day, I got lucky. I was sitting on the couch with the TV on in the background. I was reading something and stuffing my face when I heard the guy on the TV say, "The reason you are always hungry is because you're not eating the foods your body so desperately needs and is trying to get you to eat."

I stopped eating, put down whatever I was reading, sat up and paid attention.

The man on the infomercial was Dr. Joel Fuhrman. A physician who had spent over a decade studying nutrition and how specific foods affect the body. He was explaining how his eating plan worked and how, by following it, you could eat yourself healthy AND lose weight.

He went on to explain that if you don't eat foods that contain the specific nutrients your body needs to properly function each day, it will continuously send hunger signals in the hope you will eat the right things.

This is why so many of us are perpetually hungry and don't understand why.

He uses the acronym GOMBS to remember the foods one needs to eat each day. GOMBS stands for

- **G**-Greens
- **O**-Onions
- **M**-Mushrooms
- **B**-Berries
- **S**-Seeds

Intrigued, I bought his book, read it and followed the GOMBS eating plan. Meaning each day I would eat a combination of all five foods.

For example, in the morning I'd have a bowl of berries with sesame seeds and a spritz of whipped cream. Later a hamburger with mushrooms and onions. At night a green salad with grilled chicken.

IT WORKED!

After my morning dose of berries and seeds I discovered I wasn't hungry until late afternoon. I then realized that I didn't need to eat lunch and cut it out altogether. Then at dinner I could have a big hearty meal consisting of the rest of the nutrients I needed to eat that day, plus whatever I felt like eating. Except most times I became full half way through.

But here's the downside. To receive the full effect of Dr. Fuhrman's health plan, the good Doctor insists that you become a vegetarian.

Not gonna happen.

I'm going to be blunt here. My healthy eating diet plan isn't going to turn you into the godlike Adonis you were in your youth. It's not likely to cause women to throw themselves at your feet or worship you from afar.

What it will do, if you follow it, is likely prevent a heart attack or stroke or chronic digestive issues, or high blood pressure and hopefully ward off other ailments associated with middle age.

Now here's the stumbling block when it comes to most middle-aged guys and diets. And I'll put in the form of a math problem.

Old Dog + New Tricks = Not Gonna Happen.

However that isn't the end of the equation. Here's the next step:

Old Dog + New Tricks + Not Gonna Happen = Heart Attack or Stroke.

To be honest some guys look at that equation and say, "Well, so what if I keel over dead while eating a jelly donut, the kids are grown, I did my bit."

That might be true but there is still another part of the equation that these guys don't take into account and it's VERY IMPORTANT.

Old Dog + New Tricks + Ain't Gonna Happen + Heart Attack or Stroke = ***THAT GUY***

And here is why it is SO IMPORTANT that you get on board.

Because that last thing you want to become is ***THAT GUY***.

Who is ***THAT GUY***?

That Guy is the poor sap who thought that when his time came, he would simply keel over from a heart attack or a stroke and wake up poolside at God's house.

And why does he think that way? It because that's what happened to guys when he was growing up. Middle-aged men had heart attacks, strokes or aneurisms and died on the way to the hospital.

The problem is that most guys don't die like that anymore. With today's medical technology, you will likely survive heart attacks, strokes and aneurisms, and there's a better than a 50% chance you will survive a bout with cancer.

But surviving often comes with a price. You see, **_THAT GUY_** is now part of the walking wounded. The stroke or aneurism has made it difficult for him to speak. He needs a walker or wheelchair to get around. He's pale, frail and hard to look at. He wears a backpack with an oxygen tank in it. His wife clearly resents having to care for him. His kids rarely visit and when they do, they wrap it up as quickly as possible. He has tubes up his nose that you have to look at as he speaks to you. His life revolves around doctors and hospitals. He tires easily but insists he can keep up, but can't. He's slow, unsteady and always asking favors.

"I'd do it myself," he'd say. "But because of my condition…"

And what annoys you the most is that you saw this coming. In fact, everybody saw it coming. You warned him. Told him that his diet of unhealthy foods and fried crap was going to catch up with him. Told him that if he didn't get off the couch and get some exercise his body would turn against him. You tried to reason with him and he just blew you off.

"That's not going to happen to me," he'd reply dismissively.

Then, of course, it did. And now you're stuck. Because you can't abandon your buddy when things get tough, even though most of his other friends have. And so you are patient and help him with his difficulties as best you can, even though deep down you want to drop kick his stupid ass over a goal post for being so damn thoughtless and inconsiderate.

And that, my friend, is why the smart thing for you to do… is **listen.** It is why you should adjust your diet and why you should set aside a little time each day to get some exercise because the last thing on earth you want to become is ***THAT GUY!***

Here's the biggest danger to your health and well-being.

YOUR EGO.

The reason so many normal, regular guys become **_THAT GUY_** Is because of their ego.

They think going to the doctor is a sign of weakness. They have convinced themselves that strokes, heart-attacks and aneurisms happen to OTHER PEOPLE. _**AND,**_ because they have deluded themselves into thinking they have the constitution of an ox, they dismiss warnings and fail to maintain their body. The very thing that keeps them alive.

Say you owned one old car and it was the only means of transportation to get to your job. You're living pay check to paycheck, meaning that if you lose that job, it won't be long before you wind up in the street.

You would take good care of that car, wouldn't you? You'd get the oil changed, tires rotated, engine and transmission checked regularly. The whole nine yards.

You take these steps because it's an old car with a lot of mileage. And you realize that because it's old, things will need preventive maintenance, AND since you can't afford for it to breakdown, you're Johnny-on-the-spot when it comes to automobile care.

Yet too often we don't take these same preventive measures to ensure our own well-being.

Why? It's because although we age physically, *psychologically*, we stop aging in our mid-twenties. It is at that point where we establish our permanent self-image, it is the time in our lives when we decide who we are, what we like and what we want.

It is very likely the type of music you enjoyed in your mid-twenties is still the music you like today. The clothes you wear, your hair style, the type of car you like, all decided back in your twenties.

The problem is we still think our bodies are as healthy and regenerative as they were back then.

They aren't—not by a long shot.

Science has proven that we also see ourselves as younger and more attractive than we actually are. And are often startled when we see a photo or video of ourselves.

"Who's the old guy with the wrinkles," you ask.

That's the REAL you, is the answer.

And that's not a bad thing. Because seeing yourself as you actually are helps you reconnect with the fact that you are simply human. **That you are getting older and are going to require**

additional preventative maintenance to continue to live independently. To be able to do the things you enjoy and to carry out your daily obligations.

Because in this day and age, **you must never allow yourself to be perceived as old!**

This is very important, AND it isn't vanity. In the past, society viewed older people as wise and sought their council. Many famous paintings feature an old man with white hair and a long white beard surrounded by a group of attentive youth.

No longer. Older people are now viewed as out of touch and in the way. Their input in conversations is either ignored or, if acknowledged, the listeners nod condescendingly and continue on as if nothing had been said.

For example: Paul McCartney is in his seventies. But does he look it? Of course not. There's no grey in his hair, no middle age paunch, no shuffle in his step. He's still an A-list celebrity even though he's well past his prime. His secret is obvious, he doesn't look old and so he's not viewed as such.

We live in a society that is obsessed with youth and longevity. Accept the reality of your age and body condition and don't delude yourself into thinking that illness and infirmity is something that only happens to other people.

So what's our main goal here? The **MAIN GOAL** is for you to **BECOME HEALTHY**. AND to accomplish that in an easy and an acceptable manner.

That's all there is to it.

And once you get your health back, it will be easier for you to accomplish your other goals. Are you overweight? It's a lot easier to exercise when you're healthy. Depressed? Healthy people have a better positive attitude. Need to quit drinking? Fighting off cravings is less difficult when you're in good health.

Bottom line: Life is simply BETTER when you are healthy.

When I finally decided to get myself back into shape, I downloaded health and exercise books and videos and learned the usual PROVEN METHODS OF WEIGHT LOSS. All of which were guaranteed to work.

The problem was the methods were absurd. Why? Because I WANT TO ENJOY MY LIFE. I don't want to live into my nineties if for the next forty years all I am allow to eat are vegetables and various extracts and supplements of bizarre, never before heard off *natural remedies* that sound like the ingredients of a potion made by Harry Potter.

So to sum it up. What I'm about to show you are ways to strengthen your immune system so you can ward off infections and viruses, point out methods and powerful foods that will clear out the toxins that's slowing you down, strengthen your heart, lower your blood pressure as well as tricks and clever exercises that will help you lose weight without exhausting you and subjecting you to physical pain. Being healthy leads to a happier and more exciting life.

One last word so there is no misunderstanding. I am currently 20-25 pounds overweight. In addition to eating healthy foods I also occasionally enjoy drinking beer, and eating pizza and chicken wings.

I also haven't had as much as a cold in seven years.

My point is this diet will likely work because it's do-able. It does not require some drastic dietary change or some Spartan exercise regimen. But it does require you to decide to take action to get healthy, otherwise you're just wasting your time.

So don't get all fired up and overdo it. The key to success is to do a little each and every day. We're in this for the long run, not a quick sprint that peters out and garners no long term success.

If there is one sentence that sums up the most successful way to live, it's this:

Everything in moderation and for heaven's sake have some fun!

So Let's Get Started

So, how do you know if you need this book? Well the first question to ask is how often do you get sick? Are you constantly battling a cold or indigestion? Are you constipated or have diarrhea? Suffer from headaches, anxiety and acid reflux? Fatigued and depressed? Can't seem to stop eating or get enough sleep?

As mentioned earlier I am a satisfied practitioner of Dr. Fuhrman's GOMBS diet. I bought his book *Eat To Live* and it changed my life. I even sell his book on one of my websites.

But I'm not going to sell it here. Because as much as I was helped by Dr, Fuhrman's diet regimen, like most diets it goes too far by insisting that its practitioners become vegetarians.

I am not saying he isn't likely right. I'm just saying most middle-aged men will not change to a vegan diet and because they won't, they throw the baby out with the bath water and make no changes in their diet at all. And that's a mistake.

While Dr, Fuhrman's diet may very likely turn you into a finely-tuned specimen of health and fitness, my goal is to turn unhealthy habits around, rebuild your immune system and show you how to have a more active lifestyle.

Once that is accomplished and you decide to further your health and fitness regimen, by all means do so. But I believe that in order to get started you have to believe that it is something you can actually do and is something you can stick with.

Where before I was a couch potato, I now have an active lifestyle. I ice fish and go snowmobiling. I play tennis and go to concerts. And yes, I'm middle aged.

In addition, I don't want to spend my days monitoring my diet and checking my health stats. What I needed to know—and what I suspect you want to know—is what foods and exercises increase overall health?

So I made it my mission to find out.

Now a word of caution. Never make the mistake of thinking that eating healthily will prevent or eradicate any deadly disease. Although it has been proven that specific foods greatly enhance the body's ability to fight illness, don't buy into that conspiracy theory that big medicine is spending millions to keep you from finding out how to cure diseases naturally and without pharmaceuticals.

A perfect example of a health kick gone wrong is the late Steve Jobs. He received an early diagnosis of pancreatic cancer. His doctors informed him that at that early stage, surgery was his best option and he would very likely make a full recovery.

He chose instead to go the natural food and supplement route. By the time it became apparent that method wasn't working, the cancer had become terminal.

Keep that fact in mind when you read about the cancer fighting nutrients in certain foods and the heart strengthening supplements outlined in this book. Many foods do ***fight*** and ***prevent*** cancer but so far, only chemotherapy, radiation and surgery have been proven to *eradicate* it.

Which brings us to another word of caution. If you are seriously ill, morbidly obese or have complicated health restrictions like food allergies, or hypertension or afib, don't go the self-help route. What I am presenting is best suited to people who, for one reason or another, have let themselves go and need to get back into shape. They have checked with their primary care physician who has given them the OK.

Common sense and moderation are the keywords here.

Many of the foods I am going to suggest you start eating regularly fall within Dr. Fuhrman's dietary plan. However, there are many other powerful foods and by adding them to your daily intake, you can greatly vary your dietary options.

Changing Your Diet.

As mentioned earlier this isn't going to be one of those Spartan diet plans consisting of wheatgrass and tree bark. This is about trading in that tasty crap you so enjoy for alternatives that are ALMOST as tasty (yes, some minor sacrifices will be required) but they will get right to work restoring your health instead of destroying it.

Here are some things I SUGGEST you stop eating. Frozen dinners. They are filled with harsh chemical additives to prevent spoilage that builds toxicity and creates inflammation in your system. Potato chips, tacos, cheese food (not real cheese, cheese food is made from oil) soups high in sodium (most are, check the can before buying) Also avoid greasy foods, fried foods, cookies, candy, donuts and cakes, ice cream, jerky, nachos supreme and anything else smothered in cheese (again its likely oil not dairy.) All fast food from franchises, with the one exception I'll get to later.

It's been reported that many fast food and TV dinner companies spike their products with additives that actually increase your hunger. So keep away whenever possible. And if you're anything like me, you won't really want them anymore once you see the detrimental effect they have on your health and mood.

I know it sounds rough but it's not as bad as you think.

Here is what you replace your former snacks with: walnuts, cashews, raisons, grapes, (red grapes are very heart healthy) apple slices (yeah dip them in caramel, what the hell) celery, carrot slices, bread and butter pickles (Pickles works great on acid reflux) mandarin oranges, cucumber slices, low-salt pretzels, and popcorn sprinkled with parmesan cheese.

Some veggie dips are high in calories however, many are also high in vitamins and powerful nutrients like spinach dip, onion dip, dill dip, cucumber dip, horseradish dip, bean dip, avocado dip (guacamole) which is especially good at lowering cholesterol, Humus (I'm not a fan but many people seem to like it)

Just make sure it made from the actual product and not from some chemical flavoring. You might find these a little more expensive but it's worth it because you'll be eating real food that will improve your health.

Let's start with a simple example featuring a power trio. Green tea, spaghetti and tomato sauce and steamed broccoli. Not only do they ward off disease, they actively fight prostate cancer cells.

So for dinner whip up spaghetti and your favorite tomato sauce, (or create your own tomato sauce using fresh tomatoes) and while its cooking, take a strainer, fill it with cut broccoli florets and place it over a pot of boiling water. It's best to steam vegetables so they won't lose their nutrients. When it's soft, it's cooked and you can spice it up with a little seasoned salt and a squirt of lemon juice. Then toss it in with the spaghetti and tomato sauce and add a dash of cayenne pepper for added flavor and nutrients.

As for the beverage, make a cup of green tea, (if you drink regular tea, the taste isn't all that different) add some sugar, (and yes, I know processed sugar is EVIL but again MODERATION) and perhaps a squirt of lemon juice, or add a teaspoon of honey instead. Don't add milk as milk offsets green tea's healthy additives.

In the summer make a pot of green tea, let it cool then add some lemonade or orange juice to give it flavor. It not only good for you, it tastes good!

NUTS to You

Nuts are very beneficial to your overall health. Walnuts in particular. When parked in front of the TV at night, replace the potato chips with shelled walnuts. Eat a handful daily to reduce the risk of blood clots and high blood pressure. Next are raw almonds (which are a natural pain reliever) and of course, cashews which have been shown to fight oral bacteria (the type that causes tooth decay) and pistachios which can lower your cholesterol levels, ward off blood clots and help remove the sludge in you arteries.

Vitamin B-12

If you remember the cartoon character Popeye, you know that he was always getting his butt kicked by Bluto, up until he snapped open his handy can of spinach, swallowed it and instantly became a powerhouse of speed and strength. (Looking back I wonder why I never questioned why someone would carry a can of spinach in their pocket)

Anyway… B-12 works like Popeye's spinach on restoring your health. B-12 can be found in liver, red meat and eggs or you can purchase it in liquid form from your local health store and take a dropper-full every few days. It is especially good if you are having memory problems.

The Health Food Store is not Your Enemy.

Unfortunately too many middle-aged men view these places as hangouts for body building lunks looking to add more muscle and hyper sensitive vegans obsessed with having only the purest forms of nutrients entering their body.

True, you may run into those types but the advantage is that in most cases the person behind the counter knows a lot about health and especially the most effective vitamins and supplements to get you in tip top shape.

For example, each month I pick up a container of powdered magnesium and a bottle of liquid B vitamins.

For those about to drink, I salute you.

You know the health dangers of excessive drinking and I'm not your mother. However, what you may not know is that alcohol severely depletes your magnesium, potassium and omega -3. And if your magnesium levels drop too low you will experience severe muscle pain and be at an increased risk for a heart attack or stroke.

Please keep in mind that **you will be forced to change** your life style and eating habits following your first heart attack or stroke. So making small adjustments to your diet **now** may very likely keep you from having to make BIG adjustments down the road.

So if you like to knock back a few, a magnesium and an omega-3 fish supplement might be a very good idea. Also having proper magnesium levels will help ward off hangovers. As for potassium, include a few bananas in your diet each week.

Remember when it comes to your health, small changes in diet often reap big results

What to Drink to Avoid Hangovers

It's been clinically shown that it is easier for the body to process clear alcoholic beverages than deeply colored ones. Meaning you will have less a chance of a hangover if your drink vodka, gin and light rum, rather than whisky, scotch and dark rum. This does not apply to red wine versus white. Red wine is considerably better for you health wise.

I Love You Honey.

The fact that honey is highly beneficial to your health has been known since Roman times. So it is to your advantage to add it to your diet, perhaps use it to replace your white sugar use. I use it in teas and on pasta dishes made with soy sauce.

To get healthy you are going to need energy. No sense starting this if you're going to run out of steam mid-way through.

The best energy producers are Iron and Vitamin C.

Iron assists red blood cells to carry oxygen which keeps the body functions in top shape. Without iron you will experience listlessness, fatigue and malaise. Here are the best sources of Iron

- clams, mollusks, or mussels
- oysters
- beef

Here is the next best:

- cooked chicken

- canned sardines,

- cooked turkey

As for Vitamin C: People who take Vitamin C supplements of 500 mg's per day burn a third more calories during physical activity than those who don't take a Vitamin C supplement. Twice the benefit, half the work.

Another reason why most diets fail.

We have made it to adulthood. We have a family. We have learned how to survive in this difficult world. And many of those lessons didn't come easy. Making live-style changes puts us in unfamiliar territory and that makes most people uncomfortable. Familiar habits die hard.

But ask yourself, *am I thriving, or have I settled into a rut where life is happening to me instead of me making life happen?*

When I worked at corporate, I did well and after a big downsizing that I fortunately avoided, I was offered a management position that would make me responsible for an entire division.

I was 24.

Apparently it was a big honor but those more experienced suggested I turn it down because I was too young, too inexperienced and simply wasn't ready. I needed more seasoning, more time out on the road.

They were right.

I accepted the promotion anyway.

I was terrified that I would screw up something during those first few weeks. However, I was determined to succeed so I began reading books on self-improvement and building confidence. Overtime I became acclimated to my new responsibilities and soon realized that **I could do the job**.

Remember, half the battle is simply deciding once and for all **that you're going to do it.**

Once you're physically healthy you can handle the pressures as well as the exhilarations life often throws at us. When healthy, you can, as my old man used to say, "Reach down into your socks and pull out that last bit of resolve to win." However, if you've let yourself go, it may not be there when you need it.

Remember you are the family patriarch. And in times of trouble, all eyes will turn to you to take the lead. To save the day.

Ask yourself, if there were a fire, would you be able to run up the stairs, put both grandchildren over your shoulders in a fireman's carry and get them to safety? Would you be able to catch them if they had to leap from a second story window?

If at the beach and your granddaughter is swept out by an undercurrent, are you fit enough to swim out and save her?

A moderately healthy person could easily carry out those tasks

Can you imagine living with yourself if one of those scenarios **did** happen and you weren't able to do what needed to be done?

Me neither.

Let me tell you who has the best lives, who live the longest and are sought out as company.

It is people with a positive attitude. People who do things, try new things and aren't afraid to die.

If you decide to try sky-diving at age 63 and for some reason the chute doesn't open, so what? Your kids are grown, you've lived your life and at least you went out doing something exciting.

It sure beats lying in a hospital bed writhing in pain as cancer ravages your body.

So here are your options. You can live, love, laugh and be happy so when the Grim Reaper does shows up, you can smile, grab a six pack or a bottle of wine, throw your arm around him and say, "I'm ready. Let's go!"

Or you can become sedentary, eat foods that are slowly poisoning you and wind up spending the last ten years of your life on meds, and in bed slowly wasting away.

Let's Take on the Really Bad Guys First

- High Blood Pressure
- High Cholesterol
- Shortness of Breath
- Plaque in your Arteries

These are silent killers and often strike in middle age so let's look at the warning signs and what we need to do to keep from becoming victims.

High Blood Pressure: Bad news folks, there aren't any definitive warning signs that will tell if you have high blood pressure. The only way to be sure is by having it checked by a health care professional. Most medical centers and hospitals will give you a blood pressure screening for FREE, so there is no legitimate reason not to get one, especially if you are overweight or smoke. Also, don't trust those blood pressure machines in pharmacies or supermarkets because they have a high rate of inaccuracy.

A better way to keep tabs is to purchase a blood pressure tester and use it on yourself once a week. This way you get used to the test and won't be nervous at the possible results when you get a physical.

What to do if you have High Blood Pressure.

First and foremost make an appointment with your doctor. Remember they have spent **_decades_** learning their craft. So for heaven's sake don't kid yourself into thinking you know more than they do.

As men, we too often put off going to the doctor. I suppose it's our sense of pride because real men don't get sick. Real Men tough it out.

Oh, one last thing. Real Men often die young.

Practical Men, on the other hand, do what needs to be done. So get a physical every six months because early detection and diagnosis' SAVES LIVES and prevents you from becoming **_THAT GUY!_** So if your physician prescribes medication, then take it and in the meantime search for alternatives that have proven effective in lowering blood pressure. **_NOTE* always advise your health care professional before stopping ANY prescribed medication._**

Here are some proven methods:

Lose weight: DUH! You wouldn't be reading this book if that wasn't an issue. So my suggestion is to follow Dr. Fuhrman's GOMBS diet (mentioned in the first chapter) to start. There will be other weight loss tips later in this book that will help drop the extra pounds.

Walk at least 30 minutes a day: This is no secret. Everyone knows that healthy people are somewhat active people. If you're not interested in going to a gym, then mall walk. You can lose the same amount of weight by briskly walking through the mall as you can slogging outside in the rain.

Or take up golf. (Just don't use a cart)

Here's a tip to double the effectiveness of walking:

I live in a climate that is cold for the better part of the year. So to lose pounds I dress in layers to keep warm and then go outside for a 30 minute walk.

When it's cold your body has to work harder to warm the air you breathe and so it burns calories faster and more efficiently. Want to lose weight fast? Spend a lot of time out in the cold. I ice fish and go snowmobiling in the winter months and even though those activities don't require much exertion, I lose weight anyway.

But remember to dress warmly because if you get too cold and your body is using up too much energy to stay warm the brain will send out hunger signals to replace the fat stores you are burning off.

Lower your salt intake: Don't automatically add salt to your meals. Taste them first then decide just how much salt is sufficient or switch to Mrs. Dash.

I've tried it and it's not bad and comes in a variety of spices that mimic the taste of salt.

Also be very wary of frozen dinners and cold cuts. Fun foods like Pepperoni and kielbasa, salami, Virginia ham, bologna and sausage are notoriously high in sodium and sodium nitrates. So are your favorite frozen pizzas, TV dinners and pastas. **But NOT all of them**. So remember to read the ingredients and find the ones that DON'T have sodium nitrates or partially hydrogenated vegetable oil.

Make it a habit to check the amount of sodium in the frozen and canned foods you buy. In fact, it's a good idea to check the labels on all the food you're going to eat. You'll be surprised at how many dangerous chemicals and additives many of them have.

Lower your frustration levels. Stress and excess weight are the two main contributors to HBP. A proven method to lowering stress is to learn Transcendental Meditation. And no, it's not just for hippies anymore. The American Heart Association reports that Transcendental Meditation is the only form of meditation that effectively lowers blood pressure. And it also lowers anxiety levels and once practiced regularly, lowers the acidity levels in your stomach which can eliminate acid reflux.

In addition lower your caffeine intake. Specialty coffees, some sodas (such as Mountain Dew) and energy drinks (Red Bull etc.) and some processed foods have extremely high levels of caffeine, which can lead to increased stress and irritability. Replace with water or juices. Cranberry and pomegranate juices are very effective when it comes to restoring your health but often need to be cut with something because their flavors are so strong. I use carbonated water or orange juice.

Increase your magnesium and potassium levels: These have shown to be effective in lowering high blood pressure. So add these to your diet. Bananas, Apples, Spinach (not that wet stuff that comes frozen or in a can) get it fresh in a bag and use to replace lettuce on sandwiches or throw it into a salad. Beans are especially effective in restoring your health so eat bean soups like lentil or bean chili. Dark Chocolate is also good for you, but make sure it's actual dark chocolate (70% or better) not just regular chocolate with a dark color coating.

Also helpful: Acupuncture has been shown to lower HBP and listening to soft music also helps. I've had several acupuncture sessions and they were very helpful in alleviating my back and leg pain. A lot of new age music works well in bringing down stress levels.

Remember the meds the doctor prescribes for HBP is not a cure, it simply addresses the symptoms. To effectively lower blood pressure you'll have to adjust your life-style and dietary habits.

As always, baby steps. You are in this for the long haul. Small semi-regular advances in your overall health is better than some rapid weight loss regimen. People who use those quick weight loss diets almost always gain it back because it can't be maintained.

If you follow the instructions outlined in this book and begin by replacing unhealthy foods with healthy meats, fruits and vegetables, over a period of time, not only will you get used to it, you will begin to prefer it because you'll notice that you're sleeping better, feeling better, have more energy, have an increased sex drive and a positive attitude.

Now on to High Cholesterol:

Most of what was already written on combating High Blood Pressure also applies to lowering your Cholesterol levels. A handful of almonds or walnuts helps as does eating oatmeal, beans, avocados, apples, and especially salmon &

mackerel (because of their high concentration of super healthful omega -3 fatty acids) and by adding oyster mushrooms to your meals.

The enemy is Tran's fats. So how do you identify them? You check the ingredients on the package you are thinking of buying and if it lists "partially hydrogenated vegetable oil" put the package down and slowly back away.

The reality is that if you are suffering from high Cholesterol you're going to have to cut back considerably on your animal fat intake. Perhaps even cut it out altogether until you're able to get those levels back under control. As mentioned earlier, High Cholesterol is one of those conditions that people generally ignore until they have their first heart attack or stroke. And then they have to deal with the after effects for the rest of their lives.

The smartest thing you can do is address the situation now to make sure you don't become a victim.

Shortness of Breath

Simply put, if you suffering from shortness of breath or find it difficult to breathe after doing something as common as climbing a flight of stairs you need to take action NOW!

I'm not looking to scare you because it may be something easily reversed **but don't take this condition lightly.** *Because if you can't breathe, you die.*

And the quicker it's addressed the less likely it will progress into something that requires you to carry an oxygen tank around for the rest of your life.

Shortness of breath is often an indication of heart and lung disease. Or at the very least an indication that you have a serious physical condition that needs to be attended to immediately.

So let's start by talking about the elephant in the room.

Do you smoke?

If you do, you know you have to stop. You don't need me to tell you that. The evidence is overwhelming. Smoking causes heart disease, emphysema, lung cancer, throat cancer and COPD. Basically, it spends your money while lowering your lung capacity and eventually killing you.

But I enjoy it so much!

I did too. To be honest, I loved smoking. Smoked a pack and a half of Winston's for twenty years. There are few things as good as a cigarette with a cup of coffee or having one after sex.

But you probably tried quitting a couple of times and simply couldn't do it.

That was my story too. Until I learned exactly how to quit. For good. I explained this method in my book ***The Best Book on How to Start Over***.

I'm going to explain it again here because the more people who know about it, the more likely they'll pass it on to other people and help them quit too.

Here's how it works.

<u>First, you have to create a mindset where you ACCEPT the fact that you will NEVER SMOKE AGAIN.</u> Choose a day when you will stop (I chose the day after my birthday) and from the moment you wake up on that day… that's it. You will never, ever smoke again.

It is vitally important that you do this. That you accept the unchangeable fact that—starting on that day—**<u>you will never smoke again!</u>**

Because if you don't do this, you will fail. I guarantee it.

Why?

Because the majority of people who want to quit smoking sabotage their efforts by allowing exceptions, which, if they occur, will permit them to resume smoking. Usually it's some terrible event that requires them to smoke to survive this personal catastrophe. Besides they can always quit later.

Right?

Wrong!

In order to successfully quit smoking you must not allow any escape clauses to that vow. Because if you allow just one, then ANY excuse may be reasonably considered.

Here is the reality that you must accept in order to be successful: **THERE IS NO REASON GOOD ENOUGH TO RESUME SMOKING.**

NONE!

I doesn't matter if you lose your job, or your spouse, or your house, or get sick, or if a child gets sick or someone dies. It doesn't matter because…

THERE IS NO REASON GOOD ENOUGH TO RESUME SMOKING.

Why? **Because it takes five years to actually quit smoking**. And during that time something bad will likely happen.

Think back over the last five years. Anything terrible happen? If not, you're exceedingly lucky. What do you think the odds are that your lucky streak will continue unabated for another five years?

You're probably asking why five years?

Here's what happens. Most people think that once they get past the first couple of months, they're home free, smoke free, on the road to good health. They stop the Chantix, remove the patch, and toss the Nicorette gum.

What they don't realize is that there are tiny cells of nicotine floating around inside your body like tiny little time bombs. They may remain inactive for months, sometimes _**for years**_ and then just when you are absolutely convinced you'll never crave a cigarette again, one of those little nicotine cells burst, your brain recognizes it and wants that nicotine rush so bad that it sends out a smoke craving far stronger than you've ever experienced before.

It's been two, maybe three months or even years since your last cigarette, you're not prepared to handle this so you give in. You buy a pack and swear you'll throw them away after just one cigarette…

And…

Within a week you're smoking as much as ever.

This is why so many people fail. They get blind-sided by a serious cigarette craving that came out of nowhere.

I speak from experience. The first time, I quit for two years, the second, for three. I didn't make a third attempt until seven years later.

That one succeeded.

I haven't had a cigarette in twelve years.

Here's exactly how I did it.

First I created the mindset. I made up my mind that my upcoming birthday would be the last day I would ever smoke. Then I told everyone I knew about my quitting date and added that should I ever resume smoking I would pay each and every one of them fifty dollars. Think that's excessive? It's only excessive if you aren't sure you'll succeed. And if you aren't sure you'll succeed, then why attempt it in the first place? This is why creating the mindset is so important.

Second, I created a list of reasons why I was quitting smoking. I easily wrote ten very good ones on a piece of paper and placed that paper in my wallet and would read it every time I got a craving.

Third: I threw out everything related to smoking, Lighters, ashtrays, and anything else that would remind me that I was once a smoker.

Fourth: I bought several packs of Nicorette gum. Six or seven if I remember correctly. I opened them up and tore them into strips of four.

I then proceeded to place a strip literally everywhere and everyplace I might find myself. I had strips in my car, in my office desk, in my wife's car, in my daughter's car, in my neighbor's car, in my suitcases, in the pockets of all my summer clothes, in the pockets of all my winter clothes, in my wallet, in my wife's purse, in my briefcase, in my night table, in the garage, in the basement.

The point is, I made absolute sure that no matter where I went I would have immediate access to a piece of Nicorette gum.

Because this is what I learned. When a craving sneaks up on you after a long period without smoking, that craving is very strong and the longer you go without satisfying it, the more difficult it is to overcome. BUT, if you ALWAYS have a piece of Nicorette gum available, any craving can be short circuited at the beginning which will permit you to continue to the five year finish line.

Important point: Nicorette gum does NOT replace a cigarette. What it does is LOWER the cravings to a level that makes it possible for you to fight off the craving and avoid reaching for a cigarette. Cravings often last less than ten minutes. It will seem a lot longer when you're suffering from one but chew the gum and wait the ten minutes. If necessary, take a second piece, just don't give in. Remember, if it's been a decent amount of time since your last cigarette, it will likely be another long time before you get another craving. And don't forget to replace the gums you used. Always have a full supply.

This method works because every five years or so your body completely replaces all your cells, meaning physically, you're not the same person you were when you quit smoking and those little nicotine time bombs have left the building.

Plaque in your Arteries.

This is a very serious condition. If you are on daily medication, blood thinners or being treated by a cardiologist, talk to your medical professional before adding the following to your diet because the combination may affect your medication's effectiveness.

Dr. Mark Stengler (www.markstengler.com) has done extensive research into plaque removal and prevention and reports that the following vitamins, supplements and juices have demonstrated notable success in combating buildup.

1. **Tocotrienols (Vitamin E) supplements** there are two types. One good for you and one bad. So read the label and if it says d-alpha-tocopherol, buy it. If it says **dl**- alpha-tocopherol, don't buy. The addition of the l after the d means it's synthetic.

2. **Vitamin K** is found in dark leafy vegetables in the following amounts in descending order:
Kale, collard greens, spinach, Brussel sprouts, broccoli and lettuce. Since most people don't eat enough the Doctor suggests a supplement of Vitamin K2 of 150-200 micrograms. Again check with your doctor if taking blood thinning meds.

3. **Garlic extract (AGE)** available in capsule and liquid form. Those taking 4 milliliters (ml) of a brand Kyolic AGE for one year had a 66% reduction in new plaque formation compared to the group taking a placebo.

4. **Pomegranate Juice**-When it comes to getting rid of plaque this is the big gun. In

an Israeli study those patients with severe arterial plaque build-up experienced a 15% reduction after 3 months and a 35% reduction in one year after drinking only 2 ounces twice a day.

Make sure it is 100% pomegranate juice and has no added sugars. Cut the juice with an equal amount of water and drink it with meals to slow the burning of the juice's natural sugars.

An ounce of prevention is worth a pound of cure.

What most people don't understand is that the majority of foods themselves aren't bad for you. It's the packaging and preservatives that are being used to extend shelf life. That's the real danger.

Microwave popcorn. Popcorn is a great way to have a snack without all the calories and fat. However, it's dangerous health-wise in the microwaveable form.

There is a chemical in microwave popcorn called diacetyl and people who work in the factories that produce that product often contract lung problems from inhaling the gases.

A second issue is PFOA. A chemical that lines the bag. According the Dr. Oz this chemical can cause thyroid problems, high-cholesterol and bladder cancer. To avoid this issue put organic corn kernels in a plain paper bag, lay it flat in the microwave, and heat until the kernels have popped. Even better, use an air popper and avoid any chemical issues.

The next issue is that PFOA is in almost all grease resistant packaging meaning candy bars, stick butter and any food product that you don't want sticking to the wrapper. Buying some of these foods is unavoidable so, whenever possible remove these foods from the wrapper and store in a covered glass or ceramic container.

Plastic bottles and canned foods. Whenever possible purchase your foods in glass jars especially tomato products. Tomatoes are acidic and causes the chemical BPA in the can lining to leach into the food itself. BPA is also in most plastic bottle beverages.

TIP* avoid drinking from plastic bottles that have the number 7 inside the recycling triangle, or the letters PC (for polycarbonate) on the bottom.

Styrofoam cups. When used to contain hot, acidic or alcoholic beverages the chemical styrene often leaches into the liquid. The chemical styrene has been linked to nerve damage.

Nitrates

You've likely heard that Nitrates are bad for you. But what you likely didn't know was how bad. Recent studies have been gathering evidence that **nitrates in food play a big part in the sudden increase of Alzheimer's cases**.

And there's more bad news. Those same studies also indicate that type 2 diabetes may also be brought about by nitrites and nitrates.

Physically what happens is nitrosamines trigger biological low level inflammation and oxidation which is a leading cause of these conditions.

So what to do? First step: **Become a label reader,** nitrates are often found in hot dogs, sausages, bacon and cold cuts. So when shopping read the labels and select the product without the nitrates. I found several brands of hot dogs that don't have nitrites or nitrates. Same with sausage. However I was unable to find any of bacon that did not contain nitrates.

So if you really enjoy bacon, get it fresh from a butcher or slaughterhouse. And be careful with cold cuts such as turkey, ham and bologna. Many so-called healthy alternatives also contain nitrates.

And if you want to know what they are…You should probably start reading all the labels.

Quick tip: Bulk up on the vegetables, they help prevent the formation of nitrosamines in your digestive system.

Transfats

I almost expect to hear an evil scientist laugh when the word transfats is mentioned. Here's why. There are natural transfats in some meats and dairy products but usually in small amounts. The majority of transfats are, in most cases, artificially produced. They are created to make vegetable oils more solid and extend shelf life.

Here's what else they do. In even small amounts they raise your bad cholesterol level and lower your good cholesterol. And increases by 23% your risk of heart disease. In addition they're far more likely to increase your weight and lower your immunity to disease.

Transfats are more commonly found in deep fried fast foods. French fries, onion rings, commercially baked goods, doughnuts, cookies, and some margarines.

So always remember to bring this one important item with you every time you go food shopping. And what is that item? It's your reading glasses.

Most ingredients are listed in very small print to discourage you from reading them so a magnifying glass might come in handy as well.

If you see the words **partially hydrogenated vegetable oil** listed in the ingredients, it's not for you.

I this point I assume you are saying to yourself, and rather indignantly, "So what the hell am I supposed to eat!?

I understand. Remember the goal is to get you to change from your diet consisting of 75% unhealthy foods and 25% healthy foods to 75% healthy foods to 25% unhealthy foods.

To expect someone to eat 100% healthy foods all the time is unrealistic. But I believe that pointing out the inherent dangers some products can have on your health will hopefully make you a more selective shopper and a more discerning eater.

I would also like to point out that food companies only product products that people will buy. If we stop eating foods filled with unhealthy chemicals and additives, they will stop making them.

Most major companies have already seen the writing on the wall and have adjusted their product to better serve the buying public.

Most fast food restaurants now have salads and fruit cups and yogurt.

But your best bet is the buy from your local farmers market. And here's the thing. The fruits and vegetables sold at farmers markets look nowhere as appetizing as those sold in supermarkets and grocery stores.

Why? Because they haven't been genetically altered, sprayed with pesticides, dyed, acid washed, waxed etc.

They are instead good organically grown foods that promote good health, strengthen the immune system and ease digestive disorders.

During the summer and fall I do most of my food shopping there. And yes it's a little more expensive…

But so is coronary by-pass surgery.

Next: the Second Group of Troublemakers

Too often deteriorating physicality is attributed to advancing age. But that's not always true. There are several ways to eliminate or severely limit the effects of these conditions. They are:

- Toxicity
- Arthritis
- Loss of Libido

Let's start with combating toxicity. A lot of middle aged men will automatically say, "I don't have any toxicity, I'm as healthy as a horse."

Maybe, but not as much as you'd like to think.

Among other things, your liver is basically a filter. And like all filters it traps and eliminates all toxins and elements that are detrimental to your health.

However, it isn't 100% efficient especially at middle age. Over the years it has likely become a little clogged, just like any filter that is heavily used. Think of your air conditioner filter at the end of the summer or your car's oil filter after ten thousand miles.

Quite a dirty mess and considerably less effective until it's cleaned out. Especially if it had a lot of heavy filtering to do. So let's have a look at the top ten food that will detox your liver and clear out the sludge.

1. Garlic. There are few things as healthy for you as adding garlic to your meals. So buy a garlic press and use it on freshly peeled garlic and add it to your meals a minute of two before it's done cooking. Garlic turns bitter when over-cooked and doesn't need much time when pressed. And if you're worried about bad breath, simply bring a small bottle of mouthwash or mint candy with you.
2. Grapefruit. Often a main ingredient in diets, due it's cleansing qualities.
3. Beets and Carrots
4. Green tea. One of the heavy-weights that can work wonders on your health.
5. Avocados. Another powerhouse.
6. Broccoli and asparagus. Mr. Green Genes
7. Walnuts.
8. Lemon and limes. Again citrus and vitamin C
9. Cabbage. Cole slaw's main ingredient.
10. Olive oil. The only oil to use when making hamburgers, steaks, chicken or pork.

Incorporate these foods into your regular diet and you will experience a significant change in your overall health.

Loss of Libido.

The following concoction has been widely publicized over the internet as a powerful blast to the libido that some claim is as effective as Viagra. It contains all natural foods that can be cooked down to a drinkable beverage.

Here is the recipe:

Bring 10 ounces of water to a boil

Add ¼ slice of a head of cabbage

4 ounces of celery root cut into small pieces.

Cook until celery root is somewhat soft but not as soft as a boiled potato.

Let it sit 15 minutes. Do not throw out the water.

Then in a blender add the seeds of one half of a pomegranate.

On small cube of ginger

And one pinch of cinnamon

And all the contents of the pot that cooked the cabbage and celery root.

Blend on medium for 5 seconds then on high for 1 minute and 30 seconds.

Then strain through a cloth bag or use a juicer if you have one. It is important to strain as effectively as possible so only liquid is consumed.

After drinking a cupful or so, wait thirty minutes to an hour and your libido should return.

Some people swear this works so unless you have allergies or a very sensitive stomach you might want to try this before popping that little blue pill.

Arthritis Remedy:

This folk remedy goes back for generations and there are thousands claiming that it works wonders. Doctors are divided. Some say it's merely a placebo while other do admit there is some solid science behind it but want more documented evidence before prescribing it in place of pain medication.

Here's the recipe:

One pound of golden raisins.

One pint of gin.

One large glass bowl (not crystal like a punch bowl)

Large glass jar with lid.

Place the golden raisins in the glass bowl and spread them evenly on the bottom to create a flat surface

Pour the gin over the raisins until they are completely covered. If any gin is left over, cap and put away.

Place a paper towel over the bowl and let sit for 10-14 days, stirring each day to make sure all the raisins get an equal amount of gin.

After the gin is absorbed, place the raisins in the glass jar and close the lid.

Do not refrigerate.

Eat nine raisins a day. No more, no less. And no, the desired results have nothing to do with the absorbed alcohol.

You should feel relief within a week to ten days.

Choosing fruits and vegetables wisely.

Too often we forget that certain fruits and vegetables are protected from insects through the use of pesticides. These pesticides can accumulate inside our bodies and do damage so it's best to know which need to be thoroughly washed before eating or when it's best to purchase the organic version. Here's a list of those that if possible, buy the organic version or thoroughly scrub:

Apples, peppers, celery, cherries, grapes peaches, pears, potatoes, spinach, strawberries.

The following just require a light rinsing:

Asparagus, avocados, bananas, broccoli, cauliflower, corn, kiwi, onions, peas, pineapples.

It is recommended that a solution of 90% water and 10% white vinegar be used as it is the most effective at removing pesticides and wax.

Also note that all fruits and vegetables need to be washed even if they have a non-edible skin like cantaloupe and watermelon and pineapple because when you cut into them you transfer what's on the outside to the inside.

Creating the Mindset to Succeed

As said in the movie *Cool Hand Luke,* "You gonna get your mind right."

Overall this diet is very easy to follow. It only requires minor changes in eating habits and moderate exercise. As mentioned, the goal is to restore your health, not to restore the body of your youth.

And if you are looking to get back the body of your youth, you will likely be disappointed. Why? Because you're a middle-aged man and should be enjoying the perks that come with that age, not pining for the days when you were Joe Stud.

Life is an adventure. With both good and bad times. No matter what you do, or where you go, there will be times of flat-out misery that you'll have to endure.

Unfortunately, the same does not apply to good times. Good times have to be created. Good times have to be hunted done and captured.

Simply put. Good times requires effort.

Most of all, good times require a positive outlook on life. And it's very hard to have a positive outlook if you're always battling health issues, which often lead to depression.

One of the most unsettling adages ever brought to my attention was this one: ***The longer you live the more likely something terrible will happen to you.***

Horrifying, isn't it? And unfortunately very true. If you're middle-aged, then you know from experience how true this is.

Perhaps you've become unhealthy because of a tragic life-altering event. Perhaps depression has become so overwhelming you see no reason to make any effort to change anything. What's the point? What is there to live for?

If this is how you're thinking, you have suffered a massive psychological injury that has severely compromised your ability to recover and one that requires immediately medical attention.

Look at it this way. If you were hit by a truck, would you tell yourself nothing can be done and lay in the street in pain? Would you drag your broken body home and drink yourself stupid to dull the pain? Or would you go to a hospital and undergo physical therapy until you were back to normal?

My point is **psychological damage requires as much medical attention as physical damage and the longer you put it off, the more likely this injury will become permanent**. There are many professionals in the field of depression and considerable advances in medicine to help you regain the ability to think clearly and enjoy life again. Never forget that good health is a mindset as well as a physical condition.

A word of warning. Bad health leads to bad decisions. <u>Make enough mistakes and life will checkmate you.</u>

You likely already know what I'm talking about. You've seen it happen to a friend or a loved one or a parent. If you don't, here's the usual scenario.

You're in a time in your life when things are not going well. You're not eating or sleeping right and getting no exercise. Depression is becoming an issue and you're starting to drink a little more than usual. The combination of these factors leads you to make bad decisions. You foolishly cheat on your spouse, or start doing cocaine or other hard drugs. You don't pay your taxes, or start gambling, become an alcoholic or drive drunk, or start writing threatening letters to government officials, or mouth off to a cop and get arrested. Any one of these things will seriously impact your life.

And then that one mistake snowballs, you get divorced, or get audited, or get in trouble with the law. Your screw-ups are now featured on the internet. You're turned down for loans, are no longer considered for promotions, become the first to go during the next round of lay-offs. You've lost your network of friends and family, your lack of a proper diet has led to a number of physical problems, medicine is expensive and social programs are a nightmare. You're running out of money and no one to turn to for help. Remember…

Although you may be comfortable now, never forget that life is **has always been Survival of the Fittest.** Let yourself go and leave yourself unprotected and you *will* attract nature's predators.

Look around, there has never been a better time to stay alert and in good health. Lately the weather has been increasing destructive, a third of Japan was destroyed by a tsunami that also killed hundreds of thousands in south-east Asia. Hurricanes in the US have become as destructive as the bombing raids of World War 2. Drought in the western US has ended the yearly growing season.

The middle-east situation becomes more violent and horrific with each passing day. North Korea and Iran are developing nuclear weapons.

Here's another reason to stay on top of things. If you are middle-aged and have let yourself go, people are going to start avoiding you. Because they don't want to responsible should you become disabled and a burden.

Sorry if I'm sounding a little too Chicken Little with the sky is falling but I thought it important to remind you that sometimes things go very wrong, very fast and you need to be able to react quickly should an emergency arise.

So how do we build that healthy mindset? We start by exercising the mind. Playing games that require mental prowess like chess, crossword puzzles, Sudoku or watching Jeopardy. Reading or listening to self-improvement books. Learning new skills. Engaging in new hobbies. And most importantly, making new friends. Few things are as beneficial to good mental health as having a number of good friends to spend time with.

Are you introverted and don't make friends easily? Then join a chess club or cooking class or photography club. Take courses at night. This is great way to meet people who have the same interests you do. Or participate in a sport. For example: You're never too old to play golf, or go fishing.

You are at the age when you can start focusing on the things that make you happy. And finally start doing the things you couldn't do back when your main responsibility was to put the needs and well-being of your family first.

Adjustments are part of life. Most are made due to necessity. For example: Graduating from school and starting that first full time job, getting married, having your first child, buying a house, moving away from the area you grew up in. These are all things that required a change in routine.

Now that you are older and your body requires more attention, that's an adjustment you can make too.

And right now is the best time to start.

Boredom Equals Weight Gain

Other than your body sending out hunger signals when you don't eat the right foods, there are other triggers that leads to weight gain. Boredom takes the number two spot.

When we are bored we look for something to do. And eating is something, right? And we like eating, especially things that taste good. Which is why they are called comfort foods.

So the question is: **Are you hungry or just bored?**

There is a simple way to find out. Each week when I go shopping I buy a few apples and leave them in a basket on the living room coffee table.

Now here the trick. When I get a craving to eat something, I tell myself it's okay to eat anything I want—just as long as I eat an apple first.

I'm indifferent when it comes to apples. I'll eat one when I'm hungry or don't feel like cooking. Or as a quick snack on a summer day. Otherwise I can take them or leave them.

I have discovered that if I have to eat an apple, before allowing myself to eat anything else, and find I'm not at all interested in eating that apple, it tells me that I'm bored, not hungry. So instead of stuffing my face, I'll go find something to do.

It's important to recognize the difference between boredom and hunger because as we get older we often have less to do and so become bored more often.

Trigger # 3: Anxiety and Psychological Pain.

Remember Primal Scream therapy back in the 1970's? It became popular (primarily because John Lennon underwent it) and because it lowered blood pressure and lessened food cravings.

As men, we often bury our feeling because we are taught from childhood that men don't show emotion, it is considered weakness and if you show weakness you will become a victim. So when we are rejected, humiliated, beaten, fail, or lose, we're told to suck it up, press it down and walk it off.

That's what Real Men do. Which is another reason why Real Men usually die young.

Primal scream therapy also proved that we swallow our psychological pain. The bigger the pain the more food we eat to keep the pain levels down.

It's a vicious circle. And a very real one that can affect you for the rest of your life. For example, I have an anxiety disorder. There is no way of knowing whether it is genetic or psychological or an undiagnosed medical issue. But I think I know where it began:

When I was a boy I lived in New York City. And one morning, after I said goodbye to my parents, I shook and shivered all the way to school. You see, I knew I would never see my parents again and that I would be burned alive before lunchtime.

Sounds pretty crazy huh?

Except it wasn't. Because on that day in October 1962 the Russians had defied President Kennedy's orders not to ship nuclear missiles to Cuba, and had sent a fleet of armed battleships on route there. Kennedy put up a blockade and warned the Russians that is they tried to break through they would be sunk.

To which the Russians vowed to fire their nuclear warheads at New York and Washington D.C. if we did.

Although I was still a young kid in grammar school I knew exactly what was going on. I read the newspapers, I saw the documentaries of Hiroshima and Nagasaki.

I was a young boy about to die an agonizingly painful death in a matter of hours.

As for the psychological effect that day had on me, I don't know. I do know that it's been five decades since that day and I still remember how badly I shivered and shook as I entered the classroom that morning. Even at that young age I was fully aware that all those PSAs on how to survive a nuclear attack by climbing under your desk were ridiculous. Especially when the A-bomb videos showed entire brick fortresses being blown apart as easily as grass huts in a hurricane.

Probably the most frightening day of my life.

And I've been shot at.

True story.

Anyway, I'm a firm believer that *knowing what the problem is*, **is the first step in actually solving it.**

So, if you've experienced severe trauma in your life, forget that He-man bullshit and get counseling. It could be the one stumbling block that is keeping you from having and enjoying your life.

So, What's to Eat?

Not only does healthy eating make you feel better, it actually makes you look younger. Want an example? How about this?

If you're middle-aged, odds are you have greying or white hair. The reason is because the levels of copper, which produces the pigment for skin and hair, has been dropping over the years. Want to slow that process, perhaps turn back the clock? Then eat ½ cup of shiitake mushrooms with your meal. It alone provide 71% of the recommended daily intake of copper.

Did you know Cheddar cheese is good for your teeth? It kills bacteria and raises PH levels to that of a recently brushed mouth.

Eating a bowl of strawberries? Good idea only don't slice them up. Light breaks down its vitamin C.

Decided to switch to flavored or vitamin enhanced waters? Check the label before you buy. Some have as many calories as a bottle soda and caffeine.

It is an established fact that **diet sodas don't work!** Studies have shown that people who routinely drink them **actually gain weight**.

Thinking about taking nutritional supplements? There has been an investigation into the falsifying of the ingredients in health supplements. It's been discovered that many don't have ANY of the ingredients listed on the bottle. So until this is resolved, eat the actual foods that contain the nutrients whenever possible rather than popping a pill. I'm not saying don't add supplement to your diet, I'm saying do a little research to make sure the supplements you're buying are actually in there.

Eat homemade chili. It burns fat and kills harmful bacteria in the stomach. Just don't overdo it, remember your stomach isn't as efficient as it used to be, and you don't want to spend the better part of your evening camped out in the bathroom.

If you're going to eat carbs, best do it at night. Those who eat their carbs at night lose more weight than those who eat them during the day.

If you're going to watch an action/adventure movie or fast paced sport, eat BEFORE it starts. Studies have shown that people eat considerably more when watching something exciting than they do when watching something informational or comedic.

Another useful trick is serve your food on small plastic red plates. Psychologically, it looks like you're eating more food when it's on a smaller plate. Plus we've been trained from childhood that red means stop. So amazingly, people routinely eat less when served on a small red plate.

Supermarkets pipe in soft relaxing music that calms and extends the time you spend shopping. The longer you spend in a supermarket, the more likely you will buy unhealthy foods. So prepare a list beforehand and if your phone has downloaded music on it, play fast and exciting tunes to counteract.

The most effective trick is to eat a full meal before shopping. It is a proven fact that hungry people buy more.

Avoid tilapia fish. It is often the fish sold in fast food restaurants. It is farm raised on food that is not natural to its diet and it has high levels of Omega 6 which studies have shown is bad for your health. Same goes for farm fed Salmon, make sure the salmon is Wild Alaskan.

Get rid of jellies and jams. Most are just old fruit with little nutrients and smothered in sugar.

Avoid sugary cereals. Eat a small bowl of fresh fruit instead.

Best beverages? Green tea in the morning, coffee at 2pm and apple cider or any natural fruit juice at dinner.

Speaking of apple cider.

There is considerable debate regarding the healing and disease preventing abilities of taking two shots of apple cider vinegar deluded in water daily. It is also widely believed that those who ingested apple cider vinegar daily were unaffected or survived the bubonic plague back in the middle-ages.

I very much believe in its health benefits. It is also one of the vilest tasting liquids that I have ever consumed. I literally wince and shutter each time I drink it and I've drank moonshine straight from a mason jar. But as I've mentioned, I haven't been sick in 7 years (knock wood) so if you think it may help, give it a shot (but not if you're suffering from stomach ailments, in that case check with your doctor first.)

Here's another important fact to keep in mind. If you have serious heart issues you need to be under the care of a cardiologist. A strict plant only diet has been shown to reverse heart damage BUT only a qualified professional can determine the best course of action to return you to health. As stated earlier NEVER believe that a healthy diet alone can reverse serious illnesses or physical conditions.

Remember ANY decision regarding your health is a serious decision. Be as vigilant with your own health as you were with your children's when they were growing up.

What Body Type And Temperament Are You?

To get the best results with the least amount of effort requires that you learn what type of body and temperament you have.

No sense beginning a diet and exercise regimen when you don't know how your body will respond, the likelihood of it being successful, or if it is the right method in the first place.

To solve this let me introduce you to William Sheldon (1898-1977) He was a psychologist who spent the better part of his life studying body types and temperaments.

His theories are still considered the most accurate assessment even though it's been more than a half century since their first publication.

He broke it down to three basic types. They are:

Ectomorphs: naturally slim, long lean features, thin hair, sensitive to changes in temperature. Simply put, these are the skinny guys.

Mesomorphs: These are the wedge shaped muscular guys. They played sports in school, they are assertive and liked being the center of attention. They often gained weight in middle age. These are the muscular guys.

Endomorphs: Often carrying around a few extra pounds, these guys are portrayed in movies as the best friend and the guy who says "I told you so," when the Mesomorph does something stupid and gets ostracized. These are "people persons." Easy-going, fun-lovers who enjoy relaxation, food and people. These are the pudgy guys.

What Sheldon also noticed was that these three were the extremes of the type, and as such, not the norm. The majority of people consist of at least one part of another type and sometimes all three.

For example. I have long been aware that I possess two personality types that are somewhat of a tag team depending on what my needs are at the moment. I call them Stageshow Johnny and The Dullard. Stageshow Johnny is quick-witted, funny, brusk, overbearing, aggressive and eventually tiresome. He is the guy who goes snowmobiling, skiing, and plays softball. The Dullard is the opposite. He is quiet, solitary, lacks social skills and prefers to be left alone. He is the personality that goes ice-fishing, writes books, and runs my business.

On the physical side, from the waist down I am a Mesomorph. I have very muscular legs although my only lower body exercise is a brisk walk. My brother once commented that with my legs I could kick over a Volkswagen bug.

My top half however tells a very different story. I have always had an ectomorphic (skinny guy) chest and arms. Meaning I have the upper body strength of a six year old girl and the lower body strength of the Incredible Hulk.

Somehow I make it work.

So look in the mirror and see what type you are or what combination. As mentioned earlier some people are a combination all three. To zero in on your core personality take note of which personality comes to the forefront most often.

As for me, I'm usually the Dullard or the ectomorphic personality. One would have to be in order to spend countless hours at the computer writing books or running a business without going stir crazy.

However Stageshow Johnny is also an intricate part of the package. He's the aggressive part of me that strives to win in any and all competitions. He makes the Dullard finish every book he starts and he's the personality that confidently gives a lecture on the process of writing to hundreds of listeners at a time.

So, since I am aware of my body type I also realize that exercises like jogging would probably be the least useful form of exercise. Not too long ago my car broke down in the middle of nowhere and I had to walk six miles to the nearest station.

And at my age you would think my legs would have me wincing in pain the next day.

Nope. No pain, no stiffness, nada, zip, zilch.

Genetically my legs are naturally strong. However if I had to carry a ten pound bag that distance, midway my arms would have probably fallen off.

So what exercise do I use to lose weight? I chop wood. It exercises the torso and upper body and provides me with wood to heat the house. However DO NOT DO THIS WITHOUT FIRST CHECKING WITH YOUR DOCTOR. More guys drop dead shoveling snow than any other exertive action and I didn't start doing that until I had slowly brought myself back into shape using other exercises.

The ironic thing about it is that no matter how much or how long I spend chopping wood, it adds little to no muscle. Sheds the belly fat pretty well but my upper body gets more wiry than muscular.

It is important to know your body type so you know what exercises will benefit you and which ones won't.

Remember, you are what you are. No amount of exercise will turn an ectomorph (skinny guy) into a Mr. America, nor will it turn an endomorph (pudgy guy) into a skinny guy (at least not for any length of time)

So, always remember that success often depends on the information you have when you start. That you set realistic, accomplishable goals, and accept the reality that, at times, it will be difficult to continue, especially when your inner voice is telling you you're too old for this crap and to just give up.

So you've added the GOMBS to your diet but what other foods and diet tips can help shed the pounds? Well, then it's time to go shopping

How to Grocery Shop

In most cases the wife does the food shopping but for now, it's better that you do it because it's more likely you will actually eat the food if you picked it out.

To start off you should shop once each week. We're focusing on fresh foods and cutting back on the packaged and canned stuff. To avoid aggravation and long lines don't go during the times most people shop (Saturday morning and afternoon, Sunday afternoon, Thursdays and Friday nights)

Also on the day you decide to start your get healthy program, toss out or donate to the Goodwill all the unhealthy food stored in your fridge and cabinets. If the wife protests, ask her to gather the stuff she wants and to put it somewhere out of sight. Another option is for you to buy a small refrigerator for your food only. This way you won't be tempted if the missus has a Boston Crème pie dead center in the fridge.

You should note that your first shopping excursion will probably cost a bit more than your usual shopping bill. This is because it's going to take some time to figure out what foods do the best job for your particular body type.

Here's a trick I use. I avoid all fast food places because almost everything they sell is unhealthy and adds pounds. Same goes for prepackaged frozen dinners. But I do make an exception for one item at one fast food restaurant's menu and that item is Wendy's side salad.

It provides a great assortment of greens and tomatoes and peppers plus you can also add pomegranate dressing (which is great for you) and roasted pecans (also great for you).

I buy three of these a week and I add shiitake mushrooms, red onions and slivered carrots to it then pour the whole thing into a big bowl, and add the pomegranate dressing and pecans. If there isn't a Wendy's near you check out the other fast food franchises, most carry some sort of green salad and you can always add or subtract the items that best suit you. Just don't buy anything else there.

I should point out that I am NOT a veggie person. Frankly to me most vegetables taste like dirt and you'd have to put a gun to my head before I'll eat a lima bean but that Wendy's side salad is something I actually enjoy and often go for first when I get hungry.

Although I enjoy it, I don't overdo it. That is another problem with most diets. They severely restrict what foods you can eat and so after a month or so, you get tired of the same old stuff and fall back into poor eating habits. Which is why you have to mix it up and shop once a week. This way not only is the food fresh, you can buy a completely different selection and try different recipes.

The bigger the selection the more likely you will stick with it and once you start seeing results and start feeling better you'll become more committed to healthy eating.

So let's put together a food shopping list.

For the best and most proven results we'll begin with a selection of the GOMBS foods.

For Greens you have:

- String beans
- Broccoli
- Spinach (Fresh)
- Asparagus
- Romaine Lettuce
- Peas
- Peppers
- Cabbage
- Celery
- Cucumbers
- Bok Choy
- Brussel Sprouts

- Parsley
- Zucchini

I have left out a number of greens because they're difficult to find or just taste nasty.

For Onions:

- Yellow
- White
- Red
- Green Onions or Scallions
- Leeks
- Pearl Onions
- Shallots
- Vidalia

For Mushrooms:

- White Button (the most common and the one in most supermarkets and in cans)
- Shiitake
- Oyster (very heart healthy)
- Porcini
- Portobello (very meaty tasting often substituted for hamburger)

For Berries:

- Acai berry
- Goji berry

- Blackberry
- Blueberry
- Strawberry
- Boysenberry
- Cranberry
- Raspberry
- Currant
- Elderberry
- Grapes (and yes, they are berries)
- Huckleberry
- Persimmon

The acai and goji are the most powerful when it comes to restoring your health.

Here's a list of the healthiest seeds you can eat:

- Pomegranate ½ cup
- Chia seeds 1tsp
- Ground Flax seeds 2 tsps
- Pumpkin seeds ½ cup
- Sesame seeds ¼ cup
- Sunflower seeds ¼ cup
- Grape seeds 1 tbsp

The most powerful are the flax, chia, pomegranate, and grape. You can purchase ready to use flax and chia seeds in the seasoning section of your local supermarket. I us it along with my regular food seasonings.

Here's a list of other very powerful and restorative foods

Fruits:

- Apples
- Apricots
- Bananas
- Cantaloupe,
- Honeydew Melon
- Figs
- Grapefruit
- Kiwi
- Oranges
- Lemons
- Papaya
- Pears
- Peaches
- Pineapple
- Plums
- Prunes
- Mango
- Watermelon

Vegetables:

- Red, White and Sweet potatoes
- Avocados

- Garlic
- Beans
- Beets
- Olives
- Squash
- Carrots
- Corn
- Cauliflower
- Eggplant

Fish:

- Cod
- Mackerel
- Salmon
- Sardines
- Scallops
- Shrimp
- Tuna

Many of the top supermarket chains will actually cook the fish for you and package it with vegetable and rice sides. In addition to the Wendy's side salad, a couple of these in the fridge makes it possible to eat healthy when you suddenly get hungry, instead of running out to a fast food joint.

Meats:

- Beef

- Chicken
- Pork
- Turkey

It's unrealistic to expect most men to eat bland slices of chicken or turkey every single night. And to include PORK will likely have me tarred and feathered by the health gurus. But I strongly believe that it's more important to have a guy stick with the diet and occasionally eat something that isn't healthy then insist that he eat ONLY healthy foods. Because when a diet becomes drudgery and eating becomes a chore, the next stop is the local fast food place, or TV dinners and in that scenario nobody wins.

Here's a tip. When you buy hamburger meat, buy the cut with the least fat. Same goes for steak. I am aware that fat adds to meats' overall taste, but we can replace the fats with spices and marinades that will make each dish taste delicious and also be good for you.

Healthy Spices:

- Basil
- Black Pepper
- Cinnamon
- Cloves
- Dill

- Cumin
- Garlic
- Ginger
- Mustard
- Cilantro
- Sage
- Rosemary
- Thyme
- Turmeric

As for PORK, it's not good for you. You've likely seen what remains in the frying pan after you've cooked a package of bacon.

Yeah, I'm talking about that slimy thick white gunk that has congealed on the bottom and... is now in your system. It doesn't take a Harvard Professor to figure out that isn't a good thing.

My advice? Cut down as much as you can but don't be a zealot. The goal is for you to switch from having a diet of mostly **unhealthy** foods into one of mostly **healthy** foods. This is not supposed to be punishment. If you're really craving a BLT then have a BLT. But, if you have a choice of a BLT, a Tuna Club or baked Chicken Breast and you don't have isn't any real preference, go with the baked Chicken breast. It's better for you and will likely push your first major medical ailment one day further into the future.

And that's a good way to think about it. Tell yourself whenever you chose to eat something healthy instead of something unhealthy that you are doing this to postpone your first heart attack or stroke or diabetes onset one day further down the road. And most of all, it keeps you from becoming ***THAT GUY!***

Now let's talk about **Juices:**

Vegetable juice: is the number one drink (other than water) to drink to improve health. It's best to make your own with a juicer because most brand label vegetable juices are high in sodium.

Pomegranate Juice: it's filled with anti-oxidants and is one of the healthiest beverages you can drink. It's a little strong and has a lot of natural sugars so you may want to cut it with water and drink it with meals so your body can absorb it better.

Apple Juice/Cider: Remember, an apple a day? Just note eating an actual apple is even better for you

Orange Juice: But you already knew that.

Cranberry juice: Very good but beware of added sugars.

Grapefruit juice: Also good but again watch out for added sugars.

Pineapple juice: Great for digestive issues and inflammation.

Grape juice: Like apple juice, eating actual grapes is even better for you.

Tomato Juice: Sodium is often added to tomato juice so check the label and make sure it has less than 500 mgs per serving

Avoid juice "Cocktails" They often include extra sugars, syrups and other elements that cause weight gain.

Another way to lower acid reflux is to chew sugar free gum. Studies show that people who chewed gum after a meal had 37% less acid reflux.

Here is a quick health tip. Add pureed vegetables like cauliflower and zucchini to pasta dishes like mac and cheese. Most people don't notice any change in taste but ate less because the high fiber vegetables made them feel full faster.

<u>Food Preparation</u>

There is no sense denying that we are a society that, when its wants something, it wants it **now** and it wants it **easy**. That is one of the first things marketers learn when they start out in that field.

That is especially important to know when switching to a healthy diet from an unhealthy one. The reason unhealthy foods are so popular is that they are loaded with sugars and salts and at arm's reach any time, day or night.

How can anyone avoid succumbing to such a consistent temptation?

True, it isn't easy but it is doable with only a small amount of effort.

While out shopping pick up glass mason jars, waxed paper, resealable plastic food bags and resealable plastic containers with lids. Another option is to clean out used glass jars with lids and use them for storage. Glass is preferable because it doesn't contain any chemicals that can leach into the foods. Try to use waxed paper for storing freezer goods (be sure to write what it is on the outside) but if it's too much of a hassle just use the frozen plastic storage bags.

Since unhealthy food is it is always at the ready, it takes very little effort to grab a donut, a slice of chocolate cake, frozen pizza, sliders, a bag of chips and so on.

To level the playing field once you've finished shopping, take some time to prep the foods for easy access when hunger strikes. For example: set keep a sealed bag or lidded tin of mixed nuts on the coffee table. Slice up fruits like cantaloupe and watermelon and place a few slices in several glass jars then place in the fridge. Cut celery stalks into bite size pieces, and put them into glass jars. Same with baby carrots and fresh broccoli florets. When you get a hunger craving, take out one of the jars along with a container of vegetable dip (I prefer dill or spinach) and dip the celery, carrots and broccoli like you would potato chips. Or dip apples slices.

Instead of ice cream eat the watermelon, cantaloupe, mango or pineapple slices.

Instead of French fries eat a similar size bag of mixed nuts. Instead of candy, eat popcorn sprinkled with parmesan cheese or drizzled with melted dark chocolate.

Like hot? In the Asian section pick up a bag of wasabi peas. They're not only hot but they also kill bad stomach bacteria and promote good health.

As you can see there is a wide range of alternatives that taste good and are also good for you health-wise.

Here's another advantage. As you eat healthier your taste buds also become healthier and begin to prefer healthier foods and snacks, so the longer you keep away from bad foods the more you will come to enjoy foods and snacks that are healthy and good for you.

Exercise—Here's Why It's Important and Why You Shouldn't Overdo It.

Throughout our lives our bodies go through a three step process.

1. From birth to our twenties it is constantly growing and developing new cells
2. From twenties to forties it is maintaining all the cells that it has built.
3. From forties on it is discarding all cells that are no longer being used.

You've likely heard the saying, *Use it or lose it.* Well, that is a **fact.** What you don't use, **atrophies** and requires substantially more effort to get working again. Countless studies have shown that active men stay healthy longer, sleep better and have less emotional disorders.

Here's another way of looking at it.

I bought a house that hadn't been lived in for over 4 years. No power or water in all that time. After I moved in and turned on the water, all the seals burst because they had dried out from lack of use.

And to stay healthy you don't have to become some ripped body-builder. You simply have to stay active.

Guys have a tendency to get overenthusiastic about things they have decided to get into (Need I say sports?) And because guys go a bit overboard, they sometimes run into trouble. They do too much and expect too much and wind up getting bad results too often.

If you've been sedentary for a while, do not go all hell-bent-for-leather when it comes to exercise.

Slowly build up to it. And most importantly, make sure all the necessary components are in working order.

For example, how's your balance? If you said terrific, don't be so sure. Here's a test:

With a wall six inches or so to your right, stand erect and slowly lift your right leg and keep it raised for 30 seconds.

If you can't do it without losing your balance, there is likely nothing wrong with you, it's just that your sense of balance needs work.

Try it with a wall on your left and raise your left leg and see if you can stay on that one foot for 30 seconds. If not, practice until you can. If after a week to ten days you still can't do it, check with your physician, there may be an issue with your inner ear, the fluid there thickens as we get older.

Next step, walk nonstop for 30 minutes. As mentioned earlier you can walk the mall or if the weather's fine, around the block or to the store, just don't stop for 30 minutes.

If you can't so that, then you need to build up to it. So keep away from the gym or muscle strengthening exercises until you reach that 30 minute goal.

NOTE* Just a reminder, don't begin any exercise routine without first checking with your doctor. Sudden exercise after a long sedentary period can have tragic results. As mentioned earlier thousands of middle-aged men die shoveling snow each year. They never considered the possibility that they weren't physically up to it. A quick checkup before snow shoveling season would have likely saved their life.

Before getting started you need to evaluate what type of body you have and focus strengthening the areas that need improving. My lower body needs little exercise because my legs are genetically strong. Still, I walk thirty minutes a day because I enjoy walking and it gets the blood flowing. It's my upper body that needs exercise because the meat on it is not muscle but flab.

So here's what I do in between wood chopping season. I keep two five pound barbells on the table next to my recliner. While I'm watching TV, during the commercials I will take the barbells and raise them up and down over my head. Most TV shows have 10 minutes of commercials interspersed within a half hour show. So, after watching 3 half hour TV shows a night, you will have done 30 minutes of upper body exercise. And remember to start out EASY. I don't expect you to do all thirty minute your first day out. Do three minutes and see how your arms feel the next day. If fine, then do six, and so on until you reach the thirty minute mark. And start with the five pounders. It's big mistake to start out big then be unable to exercise the next day or two because your arm muscles hurt. Once the five pounders are no longer effective THEN move up to ten pounders and so on.

Next step, see how many times you can go up and down the stairs before becoming winded. When I started out I could barely do it once before needing to catch my breath. Now I do it ten times in a row without breaking a sweat.

You might be saying "What's the point?"

The point is by slowly increasing the amount you're able to accomplish each day, you will actually be able to chart your physical improvement and know for a fact that you are getting healthier.

Creating an organic garden.

This is not a prerequisite, nor is it necessary because most supermarkets have organic sections and ready to eat vegetables and fruits. However, since moderate exercise is conducive to good health, a little bending, raking, planting and weeding certainly won't hurt you. And by eating fruits and vegetables you have grown yourself, you don't need to be concerned about pesticides or what else may have gone into it.

Many of today's foods contain genetically modified organisms. GMOs for short. 60 countries have already banned or tightly restricted their sale in their countries. The entire European Union as well as Japan for example. The United States however, has not. GMO free seeds are widely available for your own garden and can be purchased at most home and garden stores.

The Next Step: Going on an Actual Diet.

I don't like the idea of diets because they force a radical change in lifestyle. In most cases they don't work over the long run and the majority of people don't understand the dangers of up and down weight gain and loss. Nor that the fat they're regaining is being stored against their vital organs.

As mentioned, I have found Dr. Joel Fuhrman's *Eat to Live* Diet to be the healthiest and the best for you physically. He has countless supporters who have experienced a new lease on life by simply following his nutritional advice.

I am one of them. His diet and healthy eating system worked wonders on me but…

I have no intention of becoming a vegetarian.

Not now, not ever.

I am a carnivore. I was born a carnivore, I have lived as a carnivore and I shall die as a carnivore.

And probably die 10 years earlier than those who strictly adhere to Dr. Fuhrman's diet plan.

So be it.

However, there is another diet that is highly effective and is recommended by doctors and dieticians alike. It is called the Mediterrasian diet. It is very healthy and isn't vegetarian.

What it does is combine the traditional foods of the Mediterranean, (Greece, Turkey, France, Italy, etc.) with those of Asia (China, Japan, Korea, Thailand, Vietnam, etc.) which gives the dieter a very large range of foods that are tasty and varied so they don't become bored.

There is even a very popular book out called ***French Women Don't Get Fat.*** It details the normal French diet, that although heavy on creams and sauces, it has no apparent effect on their health or longevity.

Studies show that those who followed the Mediterrasian diet stayed with it longer and had more long term success than any other diet plan.

Here's some facts you should take into account. The average life expectancy for the Japanese is 83 years. For the French its 81. Other Asian and Mediterranean countries also had similar life spans.

In the US the average is 77. In fact the US ranks number 30 in life expectance even though we are the wealthiest and have a highly advanced medical system.

Our problem is that we are constantly bombarded with psychologically targeted commercials that compel us to eat more fast foods and frozen dinners that are filled with dangerous chemical additives that are slowly poisoning our digestive systems! Case in point. They don't allow or strictly regulate genetically modified foods in all of the European Union and most of Asia.

In the U.S., GMOs are in as much as 80% of processed foods

It's these Frankenfoods we're eating that is causing the majority of our health problems and guys, we've got to start turning things around.

I've researched the Mediterrasian diets and they do have a very large selection of tasty foods that will restore your health and keep it that way.

The most popular is a cookbook called **The Mediterrasian Way** and it's available in most books stores and Amazon. You can have a look HERE

Now for the Wrap Up

Following my divorce I wrote a very popular book titled: **Divorce: The Middle Aged Man's Survival Guide.** And what I was most amazed to discover when researching that book was the lack of information and help for the middle-aged man.

There are tons of books that address the needs of women at any age. Diet, health, emotion, divorce, menopause, child-rearing and so on. If a woman has a problem there is a book available to address it.

When it comes to help for men, you can hear crickets chirping and we're the ones most battle weary. We're the ones the family turns to when there is trouble. We're the ones who go downstairs with a bat and risk our lives to confront a possible intruder. But unlike women we don't have a support system. And so the pressure builds and builds with no let up. This is another cause of our heart attacks and strokes. The reasons why the get fat, out of shape or drink too much.

To combat that, I wrote: ***Get Healthy: The Middle-Aged Man's Survival Guide***

Because too many middle-aged men are unaware of the effect many of the foods they are eating are having upon them.

So here's the take away from reading this book.

1. Indiana Jones was wrong! It is the age AND the mileage. A well maintained ANYTHING lasts longer than a poorly

maintained one. Accept the fact that you are getting older and so your overall health and fitness will need closer monitoring. Remember that you are not an exception to the rule. Schedule an appointment with your health care professional today and request a full physical. I know the first one is always the most uncomfortable but once it's out of the way and you start going every six months, it will get easier and easier. AND you will likely spot any potential problems BEFORE they become serious and not have to go under life changing surgery.

2. Remember the goal is to get healthy by replacing those unhealthy foods and snacks that are severely taxing and damaging your aging system and internal organs with those that can restore, rebuild and replenish them.

3. Read the labels. Always bring your reading glasses when you go shopping. Remember that **Nitrites, Nitrates, BPAs, PFOAs** and **partially hydrogenated vegetable oil** are particularly damaging to your health. Avoid buying any foods that contain them and omit them from your diet whenever possible.

4. Don't be a zealot but don't be push-over either. Reality dictates that once in a while you will want to eat something that is unhealthy. So eat it. But then regroup and

become even more determined to stick to your healthy eating plan.

5. Always keep in mind that the very last thing you want is to become ***THAT GUY!*** A burden to your wife, family and friends. Nobody wants the added work of taking care of you, cleaning up after you, wheeling you around, or the added expense of your prescriptions. Especially when all that is required to turn your health around is to make small reasonable adjustments to your eating habits.

Foods that I eat daily:
Here's how you get started.

For Breakfast:

Monday: Two slices of cinnamon toast topped with blueberries and two teaspoons of ground flaxseeds, real maple syrup and a spritz of whipped cream and a cup of coffee.

Tuesday: Cantaloupe and watermelon slices with walnuts and one slice of buttered toast and a cup of green tea with one teaspoon sugar.

Wednesday: Two sunny side up eggs with two natural sausage links and a cup of baked beans. A cup of green tea.

Thursday: Cinnamon apple sauce, two hard boiled eggs and a cup of red grapes. A cup of coffee.

Friday: A bowl of natural oatmeal topped with raisins and brown sugar (watch out for additives) and a small can of mandarin oranges. A cup of green tea.

Saturday: Two slices of toast with butter and cinnamon sugar, a cup of cherries and small baked potato with a little sour cream, pinch of salt and pepper. A small glass of pomegranate juice cut with sparkling water.

Sunday: A toasted bagel with one slice of cheddar cheese, a sliced tomato seasoned with cracked pepper, two slices of bacon, lettuce and mayo.

Do you see how doable this is? All of the foods listed above aren't some strange combo you've never heard of before. These are foods you eat on a regular basis anyway, in this case however, we're just eliminating the stuff that's bad for you.

And if you're concerned about losing weight, don't be. When you eat healthy, your body does the work of eliminating unneeded weight by decreasing your appetite and increasing your stamina and energy levels.

For Lunch:

Most days I skip lunch because I've been eating the GOMBS foods each day and I don't get hungry until four or five in the late afternoon. Until you reach that point, here are some suggestions for lunch.

Monday: A buffalo burger with mushrooms onions, lettuce and tomato with ketchup. A side of steamed string beans with sliced almonds, onions and garlic. A cup of green tea.

*Note: <u>Buffalo meat is leaner and more nutritious than regular cow meat.</u> Substitute it whenever possible. It even tastes better.

Tuesday: Peanut butter and banana sandwich. A bag of chemical free popcorn and a bowl of homemade soup. A glass of apple cider.

Wednesday: Chicken salad sandwich with lettuce and tomato on seeded rye. Cup of tomato soup and a cup of coffee.

Thursday: Turkey sandwich with cranberry sauce with guacamole spread on whole wheat. A bag of cashews and a cup of green tea.

Friday: Wendy's side salad with two pieces of grilled chicken and a glass of chocolate milk.

Saturday: Tuna fish salad, with black olives, onions, sliced almonds and roasted sesame seeds on sourdough bread. White grapes and green tea.

Sunday: Wendy's side salad with added slices of portabella mushroom and ground flax seeds with pomegranate dressing and pecans. Small bowl of chili.

The most important thing to remember is that we are replacing unhealthy foods with healthy ones. And yes it requires a little effort BUT, never forget that it only takes one heart attack or stroke

and your diet will permanently change whether you like the foods or not. So basically what we're doing here is keeping two steps ahead of the avalanche.

For Dinner:

Monday: Steamed Haddock with roasted vegetables. I purchase this from my local supermarket along with two other seafood meals with added sides. As mentioned earlier having seafood meals prepared on site by your local supermarket chefs will garner you a great meal without any of the dangerous additives that come with many frozen dinners. A glass of red wine.

Tuesday: Steak with pearl onions, sautéed mushrooms, mashed potatoes, string beans with slivered almonds and a lite beer.

Wednesday: Spaghetti with tomato sauce, steamed broccoli, red peppers, onions and mushrooms. Plus a Wendy's side salad with pomegranate dressing and pecans and a glass of fresh lemonade.

Thursday: Second Seafood dinner purchased from supermarket. Just take it out of the fridge, microwave it and you have dinner ready. And it's delicious too. Just remember to check the expiration date. Since there aren't any preservatives added, it won't remain fresh beyond a couple of days.

Friday: Meatloaf with buffalo meat and ground pork. Follow standard meatloaf recipe. Add a serving of baked beans and a cucumber salad with lite Italian dressing. Juice of your choice.

Saturday: Big Grilled Chicken salad with grape tomatoes, cucumbers, spinach, slivered carrots, cashews, scallions and fresh broccoli florets. Your choice of dressing with a glass of red wine.

Sunday: Homemade pizza with whatever toppings you want but with as few processed foods as possible (pepperoni, ham, or other cold cuts) fresh sausage, chicken, lean red meat are fine as is any vegetable or fruit.

Important Note* You may hate all the foods I pointed out and that's fine. We're all different. The most important thing to remember is to eat the foods that properly fuel your system— GOMBS, stay away from anything that has Nitrites, Nitrates, or partially hydrogenated vegetable oil. Always check the labels on any food you buy to make sure you're not slowly poisoning yourself with chemical additives or genetically modified foods.

And lastly, remember what I said about becoming ***THAT GUY.*** There are no do-overs, no second chances once that happens. I'm sure you'd want to dance at your children's weddings. Play catch with your grandson, walk your daughter down the aisle. Enjoy the golden years of your retirement…

For a healthy man, that's a lot of happy things to look forward to.

THAT GUY however, will likely miss them all.

Thanks for reading Get Healthy-The Middle-Aged Man's Survival Guide. If you would like to leave a review go to www.amazon.com and in the search box type in   Zackary Richards

Other books in this series is Divorce-The Middle-Aged Man's Survival Guide

www.ingramcontent.com/pod-product-compliance
Lightning Source LLC
Chambersburg PA
CBHW050537280326
41933CB00011B/1616